DREAD
DISEASES

DREAD DISEASES

BY MARIANNE AND MARY-ALICE TULLY

A First Book
Franklin Watts
New York / London / 1978

To Jimmy on his way
to Sierra Leone

Cover design by Ginger Giles
Diagrams by Vantage Art, Inc.

Photographs courtesy of:

World Health Organization: p. 6;
Center for Disease Control, Atlanta, Ga.: p. 11;
Grolier Picture Library: p. 24;
Medic Alert Foundation International: p. 36;
American Cancer Society: pp. 44, 46.

Library of Congress Cataloging in Publication Data

Tully, Marianne.
　　Dread diseases.

　　(A First book)
　　Bibliography: p.
　　Includes index.
　　SUMMARY: Discusses symptoms and treatment
of diseases that seriously threaten human life, in-
cluding smallpox, rabies, venereal diseases, genetic
and heart diseases, diabetes, multiple sclerosis, and
cancer.
　　1. Diseases—Juvenile literature. [1. Diseases] I.
Tully, Mary-Alice, joint author. II. Title.
RB151.T8　　　　　　616　　　　　　78-4658
ISBN 0-531-01406-1

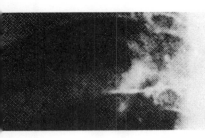

CONTENTS

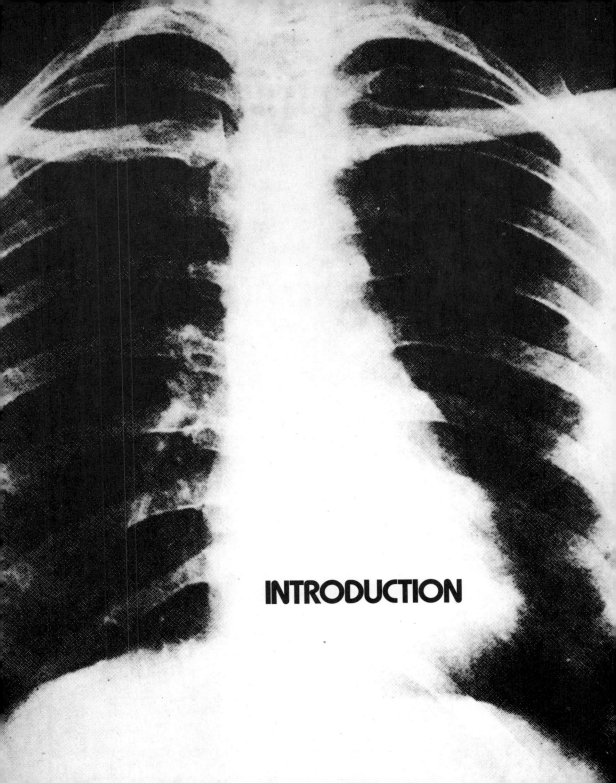

INTRODUCTION

Laughing, playing tag with your friends, sleeping soundly, stretching your whole body with a yawn, feeling hungry, sinking your teeth into an ice-cold piece of watermelon, riding a bike downhill, splashing in water, having sparkling eyes and clear skin—when all is in perfect running order, you can feel that special zing. We call it good health.

Good health is the balanced state of the body. Even though you are constantly attacked by **germs** and other stressful forces, your bodies in good health are able to throw them off. Ill health, on the other hand, results when the functions of the body are not in balance for various reasons. Then your body is not as able to protect itself from attack. The body reacts to the attack. You feel sick: tired out, hot, uncomfortable, chilly, congested, in pain. You look sick: pale or flushed face, rash on skin, swelling, coated tongue, dull eyes, weight loss. Depending upon the strength and presence of these and other **symptoms,** doctors are able to determine which illness a person has.

A disease may affect the whole body or any of its parts. Each disease has a specific cause, although in the case of some the cause is still not known. Tiny **organisms**, like **bacteria** and **viruses,** may infect the body from the outside, and cause what are called the **infectious diseases**. Other diseases involve a part of the body that does not work right. The problem may be there at birth, or may be acquired later in life. These are the **non-infectious diseases.**

The diseases that are described in this book were chosen for many reasons. All of them are called "dread diseases" because they are or were a serious threat to human life. Some were chosen for their historical importance, for example, **smallpox** and **rabies.** Some were chosen because they are the number-one killers today. **Heart disease, cancer** and **diabetes** lead this list. Others are the serious diseases that are passed from parent to child. Still others, for example, **multiple sclerosis**, were chosen because they are still so mysterious—the cause or cure is still unknown. Finally, **venereal diseases** were chosen because their spread in the last twenty-five years has reached almost **epidemic** proportions.

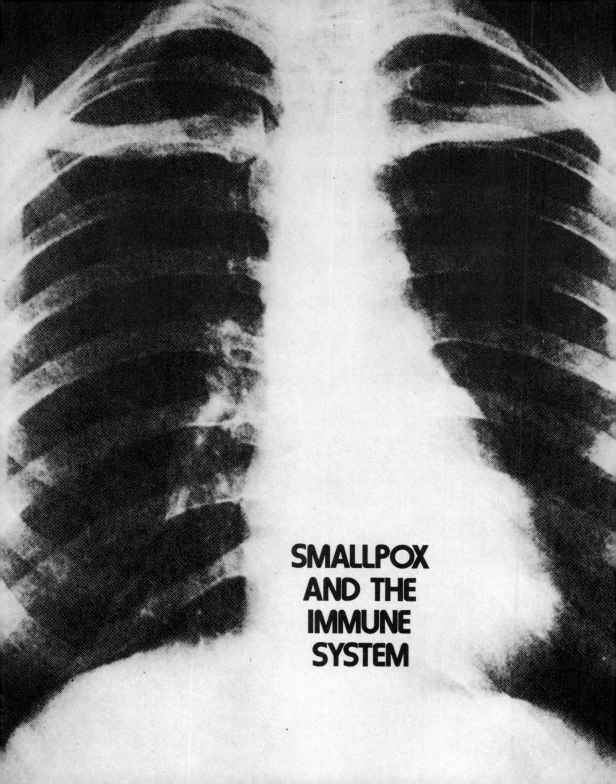

SMALLPOX
AND THE
IMMUNE
SYSTEM

In the past the most dreaded diseases were usually the infectious diseases. Diseases such as the **black death** wiped out entire populations. Most of these diseases have been conquered. **Vaccines** have been developed. These conquests have not come quickly or easily. It took the efforts of a great number of dedicated men and women.

Edward Jenner was one of these people. Through his keen powers of observation, he discovered a vaccine for smallpox. In the late eighteenth century, this English country doctor noticed that dairymaids who had been infected with the mild **cowpox** never died from smallpox. He scraped off some of the **pus** from the sores of a dairymaid infected with cowpox. He then applied the pus to a small scratch on the skin of an eight-year-old boy. This procedure is called **inoculation.** He then tried to inoculate the boy with smallpox. As in the case of the dairymaids, the infection did not take hold. This process of inoculation with cowpox he called **vaccination,** from the Latin word *vaccinus,* which means "of or from a cow." Pasteur, the famous nineteenth-century French chemist, borrowed the term and used it for any inoculation that prevents disease.

Not until 1950 was a potent dried vaccine for smallpox developed that could be shipped to the four corners of the world. Previously, the vaccine only worked if the cowpox virus was still alive. This discovery prompted the **World Health Organization** in 1967 to launch a major campaign to eliminate smallpox completely. It has been quite successful. In the United States and the United Kingdom children no longer receive the smallpox vaccine automatically, since the threat is so slight. The few cases that have occurred recently were limited to remote areas of Ethiopia.

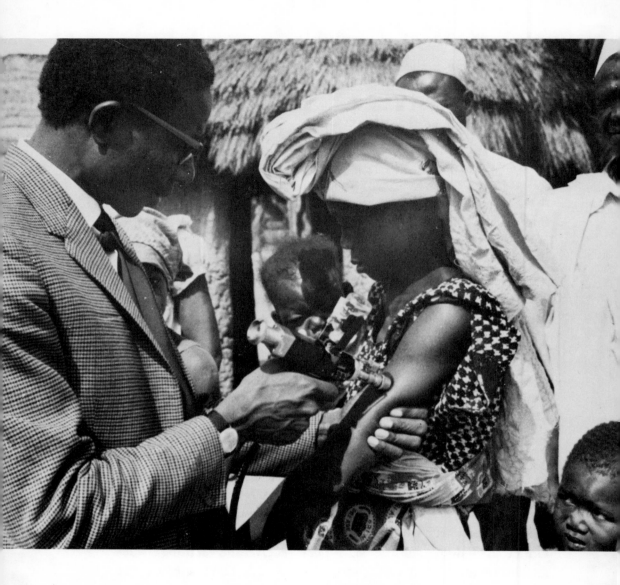

Vaccination is quick and simple
with this jet injector gun.

If no other cases are reported for a number of years, smallpox will no longer exist on the face of the earth. This will mark the first such achievement in the history of medicine.

THE IMMUNE SYSTEM

Such an achievement would be impossible without the scientist's silent partner—the body's **immune system.** Of what value would a vaccine be without the body's ability to recognize foreign invaders and to manufacture weapons against them. This ability to resist infection is called **immunity.** The immune system is complicated but basically it consists of special white blood cells and special **proteins.** The cells and proteins travel in the blood. The special cells engulf foreign invaders. The proteins called **antibodies** are able to recognize foreign substances called **antigens** and stick to them. This makes an **antibody-antigen complex.** Other proteins called **complement** are then able to combine with the antibody-antigen complex and destroy the foreign invaders.

For every type of disease or for every type of antigen a special type of antibody has to be made by the body. This places certain limits on the immune system. If a disease-producing organism attacks, and the body doesn't have antibodies for that disease on hand, the infection spreads faster than the body can make antibodies. This is why vaccinations are so helpful. The microorganisms contained in a vaccine are dead, weakened, or, as in the case of smallpox vaccine, similar to the disease-producing organism. They are not strong enough to cause the disease. But, they are still recognized as foreign, so antibodies are made against them. Then, when strong forms of the microorganism attack, the body has ready-made weapons to fight them off. This is called **active immunity.**

There is another kind of immunity. This immunity is acquired when a doctor gives a patient the antibodies themselves. These antibodies are obtained from the blood **serum** of animals or humans who were previously exposed to the disease. Since the person did not make the antibodies, it is called **passive immunity.** The borrowed antibodies are soon broken down in the blood. Passive immunity does not last as long and is not as effective as the active immunity that results from a vaccine.

Scientists are developing new vaccines all the time. They are working on one for **hepatitis,** a **viral** disease that can cause severe damage to the liver. All that has been available until now has been the antibody serum. Vaccine tests on humans were started in 1975, and the results have been promising. However, it will take years of further testing before this vaccine is available for general use. Developing vaccines is not an easy task. The ideal vaccine is one that provides immunity against a disease without causing harmful side effects. The **swine flu** vaccine project was sponsored by the United States government in 1976–77. Because of the possible relationship between a particular type of **paralysis** and the vaccination, this nationwide project was halted.

It takes many years of research and testing to work potential problems out just as it did for the vaccines for **measles** and **polio.** Children are now automatically vaccinated for **mumps,** measles (rubeola), German measles **(rubella), diphtheria, whooping cough** (pertussis), **tetanus,** and polio. The great fear that these diseases once caused is almost forgotten. In fact, many people neglect to get the vaccinations at all, and because of this, small outbreaks of these diseases still occur. Unlike the smallpox virus, the organisms that cause diphtheria, measles, and polio are still lurking. They are still a threat.

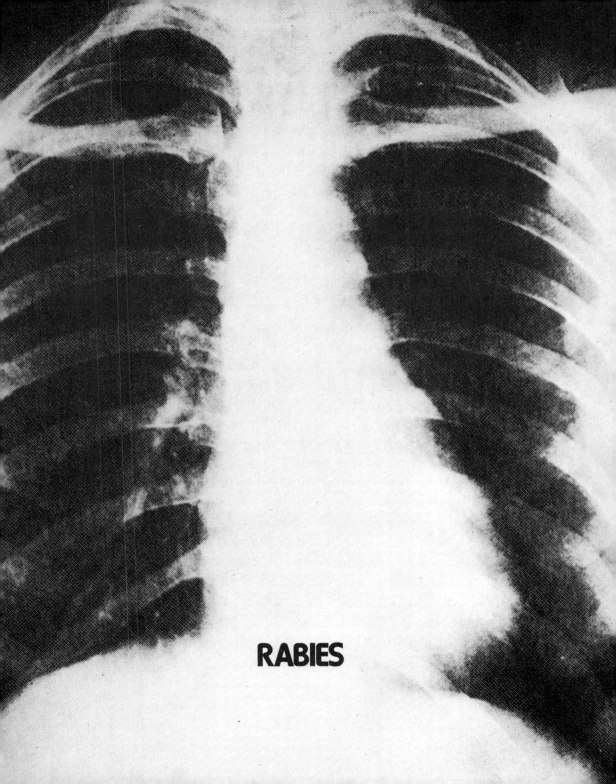

RABIES

"Mad dog! Mad dog!" That is the cry that sent shivers down the back of Louis Pasteur. He grew up hearing the bloodcurdling howls of rabid dogs. These dogs, in their vicious state, were prone to attack and bite people and pass on the disease of rabies to them. Throughout his life, Pasteur was haunted by the terrible sight of people dying of this disease. It was this memory perhaps that sent him searching for the cause and cure of rabies. Though he didn't find the tiny virus or an actual cure, he was successful in developing a vaccine for rabies in 1885.

RABIES SYMPTOMS

Rabies is a disease that is found in mammals. It is spread most commonly by the bite of mammals such as dogs, cats, foxes, rats, and vampire bats. The rabies virus is contained in the animal's saliva. The saliva infects the bite wound. The virus then attacks the **central nervous system** and symptoms begin to appear. The time between exposure and the appearance of symptoms is called the **incubation period.** In humans the incubation period of rabies usually lasts from two to eight weeks, but can be as short as nine days and as long as two years. The time depends upon the location and extent of the bite: the closer to the brain, the shorter the incubation period.

After the incubation period the disease goes through two or three more stages. In the first stage, there is usually numbness and tingling at the site of the wound. The person may be sensitive to bright lights, noise, and temperature changes. He or she may experience fever, headache, nausea, fatigue, or mental depression. Sometimes the person has trouble sleeping and has nightmares. Drooling and perspiring may occur. This stage usually lasts from one to nine days.

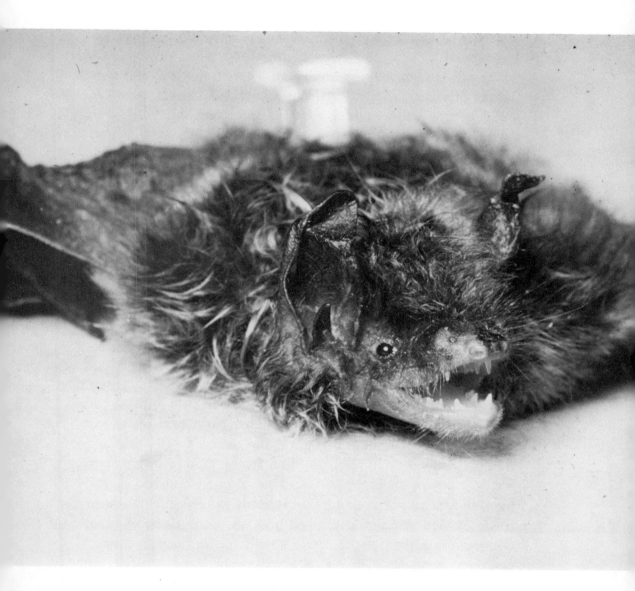

A rabid bat

The second stage is known as the excitement phase or "furious rabies." It is to this stage that we owe a second name by which rabies is known, **hydrophobia.** This means fear of water. During this stage, the very sight or sound of water causes in the victim severe spasms of the muscles used for swallowing. The spasms send the person into a state of frenzy. This stage is also marked by excessive drooling, spitting, insane actions, and convulsions. Periods of calm alternate with these periods of frenzy. Stage two lasts from one to three days. Most people die at this stage.

If they survive, the muscle spasms stop and they enter the third stage or the "dumb rabies." All of the muscles of the body gradually become paralyzed. A **coma** results and then, after six to eighteen hours, death occurs.

One reason rabies is such an extremely terrifying disease is that the person passes through the three stages with complete consciousness. Close to 100 percent of the cases of rabies result in death. This is why prevention is so important.

TREATMENT

If a person has been bitten by an animal suspected of having rabies, the wound should be thoroughly cleansed with soap and water. It should be allowed to bleed freely. Within seventy-two hours, a doctor should inject a serum of rabies antibodies into the skin around the wound. Until recently the Pasteur treatment was used. The vaccine, developed from the brain **tissue** of rabid dogs, was injected into the person's belly for fourteen to twenty-one days in a row. This was a terrible experience. There were often bad side effects from the brain tissue vaccine.

There has been a major breakthrough in the development of a new rabies vaccine. This vaccine does not cause the harmful side effects of Pasteur's treatment, since it is made from tissue other than nervous tissue. Also, this vaccine requires less than six injections. It was tested in Iran during 1975–76 with excellent results.

The best way of stopping the threat of rabies in people is to prevent and control the disease in animals. In countries where rabies is present, household pets should be periodically vaccinated for rabies. Any animal that appears sick should be avoided and reported to the health authorities. Some countries, such as the United Kingdom, quarantine all animals entering the country for six months, and thus have remained free of rabies. But it only takes one smuggled animal with rabies to bring the disease in.

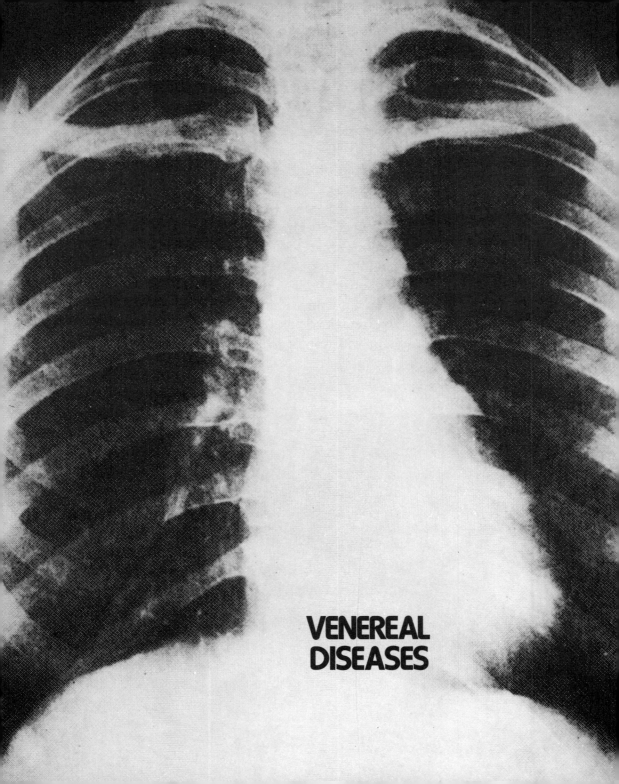

VENEREAL DISEASES

Venereal disease (VD) is the number-one epidemic in the United States and one of the most epidemic diseases in the United Kingdom. The name "venereal" comes from Venus, the Roman goddess of love. This name is used because an infected person spreads the disease through sexual contact. There are five different types of VD, but the major ones are **syphilis** and **gonorrhea.**

VD has been known to civilization from earliest times. Certain diseases described in the Bible and other ancient literature may have been venereal diseases. Both gonorrhea and syphilis had major outbreaks at the end of the fifteenth century in Spain, France, Italy, Germany, and part of what is now Russia. Often people were afflicted with both **infections.** This led early scientists to think that they were part of the same disease. Not until the **microbes** that caused each infection were identified by Benjamin Bell in Scotland in 1793 were the diseases considered separate. Syphilis is caused by a spiral-shaped microbe called a **spirochete.** Gonorrhea is caused by a round bacterium called a **gonococcus.**

SYPHILIS

There are three stages of syphilis. The first stage is marked by the appearance of a painless sore called a **chancre.** This sore is found in the **genital area** in 90 percent of the cases. During this stage the disease is highly **contagious.** The chancre goes away without treatment in four to six weeks. The disease is then considered to be in its second stage. The spirochete is now traveling in the bloodstream. During this stage, it is possible for pregnant women with syphilis to pass the disease to a developing fetus through the blood supply. All pregnant women are routinely tested for syphilis to prevent this from happening. As the spirochete travels in the blood, generalized symptoms appear, such as fever, loss of appetite, tiredness, a rash on the body, and sores on

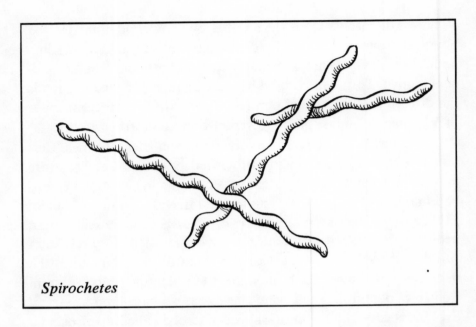

Spirochetes

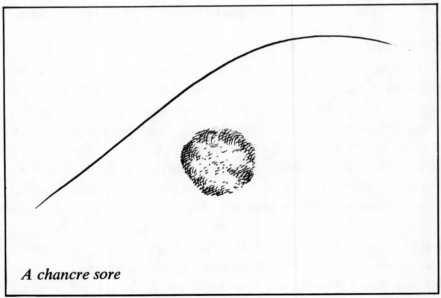

A chancre sore

the **mucous membranes.** The rash and sores are teaming with the spirochete that caused the disease. Now it is even more contagious. These symptoms also disappear in two to six weeks. The disease then becomes **latent,** or inactive, and it shows no symptoms at all. At this time it is rarely contagious. Finally, the third stage makes its appearance after fifteen to twenty years. The main symptom is the formation inside the body of horrible sores called **gumma.** These gumma eventually destroy all tissue, especially the heart, blood vessels, and the tissues of the nervous system.

GONORRHEA

The symptoms of gonorrhea are quite different from those of syphilis. In males, gonorrhea is immediately recognized by painful urination with a thick mucous discharge. Females may experience these same symptoms. However, 80 percent of the women

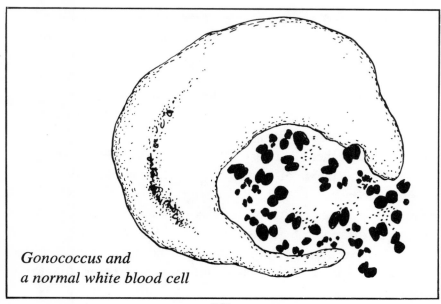

*Gonococcus and
a normal white blood cell*

infected have no symptoms. This is one of the dangerous things about gonorrhea. The disease can be spreading within the body and can be spread to other people without the victim's knowledge. The disease then inflames the genital and **pelvic organs** of both males and females and can lead to sterility. Sterility is the inability to have children.

Gonorrhea can be passed from mother to child in the process of birth. As the baby travels through the mother's infected birth canal (vagina), the baby has direct contact with the gonococcus bacteria found there. The infection mainly affects the eyes of the baby. If not treated with **antibiotics,** blindness may result. To prevent this, pregnant women in the United States are routinely tested for gonorrhea and, immediately after birth, babies receive eyedrops to kill the gonococcus organism.

TREATMENT

Both syphilis and gonorrhea are easily cured by antibiotics such as **penicillin** or **tetracycline.** People do not build up an immunity to these diseases. They can be caught again and again if the person is exposed to them. What has worried public health doctors so much is that new strains of gonorrhea are developing that are resistant to penicillin and other antibiotics. Larger doses are needed to kill these strains.

Although there is a cure for VD, people do not always seek the cure. The personal nature of the disease may make some people uncomfortable about seeking medical help. Or, some people may think that the disease is gone just because the early symptoms disappear by themselves. Finally, some people may refuse to believe that they could ever get the disease, even if they have been exposed to it. These attitudes are being fought by public health officials.

[18]

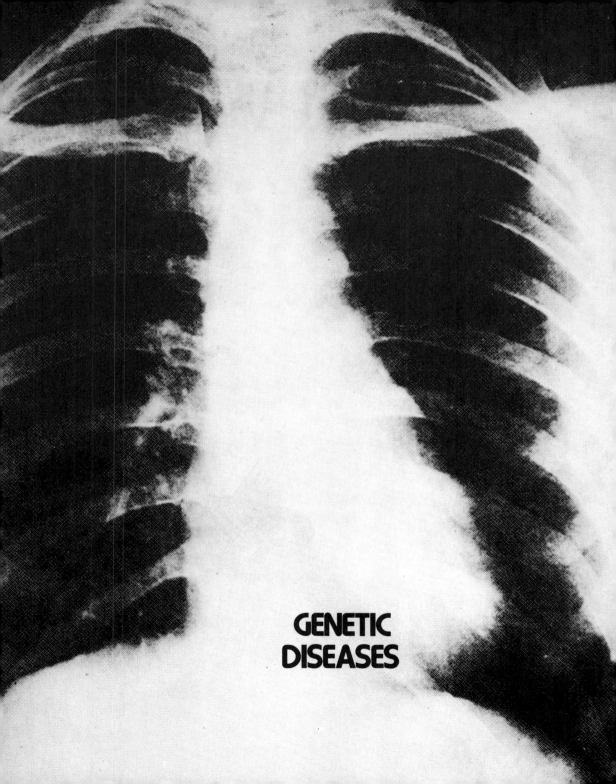

GENETIC
DISEASES

Three-year-old Brenda had been sickly since she was a baby. She was a thin, quiet child. One morning she woke up crying. She was in great pain. Her mother remembered that Brenda seemed as if she were coming down with a virus the day before. Now, Brenda's stomach felt hard. She had a fever. She was twisting and turning in an effort to get away from the pain. Her parents took her right to the hospital. They feared that she was having an attack of appendicitis.

After many tests, the doctors discovered that Brenda had **sickle cell disease.** She was born with it, but this was the first flare-up, or "sickle cell crisis." She inherited this disease from her parents. It is caused by a pair of abnormal **genes.**

GENETICS

A gene is a unit of **heredity.** All of your main physical **traits** are determined by the genes that you received from your parents. The gene is a section of a **chromosome.** Twenty-three pairs of these chromosomes are found in each human body cell. Half of your chromosomes came from your father and half from your mother. The chromosomes are composed mostly of **DNA** (*d*eoxyribo*n*ucleic *a*cid). The DNA provides the pattern in which each organism may grow and develop. If a change occurs in the DNA pattern or gene, it is called a **mutation.**

ORIGIN

Sickle cell disease began as a mutation. The original mutation occurred over one thousand years ago in Central Africa. It has been passed on from one generation to the next until the present time. Now about 10 percent of all American blacks carry at least a single gene for sickle cell.

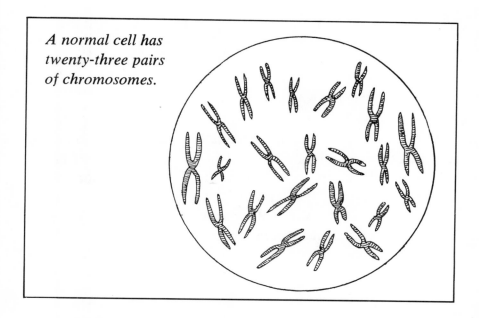

A normal cell has twenty-three pairs of chromosomes.

SICKLE CELL TRAIT

When people carry only a single gene for sickle cell, instead of the full pair, they have the **sickle cell trait.** These **carriers** usually have no symptoms of the disease but they can pass the gene on to their children. The reason why they do not have the disease itself is because the sickle cell gene is a weak or **recessive gene.** Both genes of a pair must be present for the recessive quality to appear in an organism. A **dominant gene** on the other hand is a strong gene. A trait produced by a dominant gene is obvious in the organism even when only one of the pair is present.

If a male and female carrier of the sickle cell trait have a baby, there is a 25 percent chance that the baby will have both recessive genes (one from each parent) and have the sickle cell disease. The baby has a 50 percent chance of getting only one recessive gene and therefore of carrying the sickle cell trait. And there is a 25 percent chance that the baby would receive no recessive gene for sickle cell at all and be perfectly clear of the disease.

SICKLE CELL DISEASE

Directed by the pair of sickle cell genes in the nucleus of each cell, the body makes some **hemoglobin** that has one chemical substituted for another. Hemoglobin is a protein found in the red blood cells. When the normal amount of oxygen is not present in the bloodstream, the mutant hemoglobin molecule changes shape and distorts the shape of the entire red blood cell. The cells look like sickles instead of the normal disc shape. This action of sickling usually begins in some localized area of the body, like

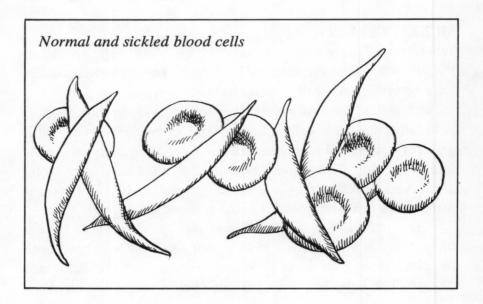

Normal and sickled blood cells

the stomach or the joints of the legs. The abnormal sickled cells also tend to clump together or to stick to the sides of the blood vessels. This causes a blockage. Pain and **inflammation** follow. This causes the sickle cell crisis.

The sickled red blood cells have a shorter life than the normal ones, so that **anemia** commonly develops. Anemia is a decrease in the normal number of red blood cells. This results in less oxygen being carried by the red blood cells to all parts of the body. Severe anemia may cause sudden death in a young child.

Sickle cell disease is marked by possible problems in every area of the body—heart, lungs, liver, and kidneys. Doctors have no cure for sickle cell disease and can only relieve the symptoms. There is now an emphasis on testing large groups of people to determine if they carry the trait. The testing of the general population is called screening. With adequate screening and good general care, the life expectancy of people with sickle cell disease has been greatly increased and they have been able to live more normal lives.

TAY-SACHS DISEASE

Another **genetic** disease is **Tay-Sachs disease.** It is most commonly found in Jewish people who have ancestors from Central and Eastern Europe. Like sickle cell disease, Tay-Sachs is caused by a single recessive gene. A baby born with Tay-Sachs disease seems perfectly normal at birth. But, by the age of six months, things start to change. The baby's development begins to slow down. At first, the parents are not even aware of it. What is happening within the baby's body is this. The mutated gene pair, which the child inherited from both parents, makes the body store too much of a fatty material in the cells, particularly the

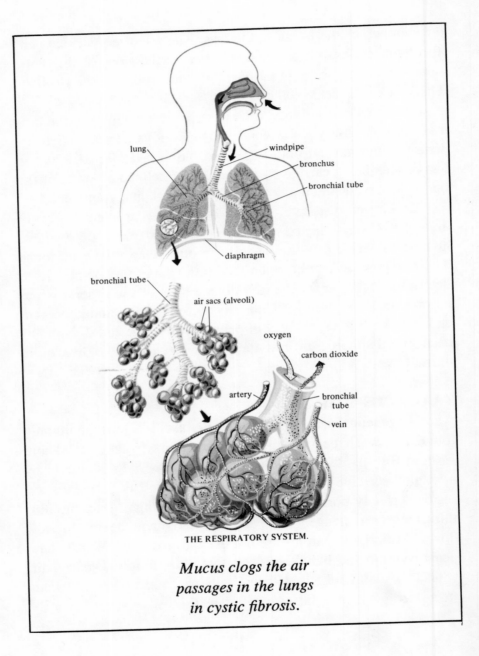

THE RESPIRATORY SYSTEM.

Mucus clogs the air passages in the lungs in cystic fibrosis.

brain cells and other nerve tissue. This makes the brain cells swell up, burst open, and die. Gradually, the infant loses whatever motor abilities it had already developed. The child becomes increasingly less able to sit up, to roll over, to reach out, and to respond. Gradually too, the brain does not function as it should and the child becomes mentally retarded. Death usually occurs at the age of two or three. There is no treatment or cure for Tay-Sachs disease.

CYSTIC FIBROSIS

Cystic fibrosis is another disease that is caused by a recessive gene. One baby in every 1,600 births is born with this disease. It occurs mostly in Caucasian races and is very rare in blacks. When a child is born with the trait from each parent, the glands of his or her body that make mucus, saliva, and sweat are affected. It is still not known why widespread changes occur in these glands. A gluey, sticky mucus clogs the air passages in the lungs making breathing difficult. Respiratory infections are a **chronic** problem. Cystic fibrosis (CF) is the most serious lung problem affecting children in the United States and Europe today.

Thick secretions may also block the **pancreas.** This prevents the gland from secreting the necessary digestive juices. The child will have trouble digesting food and may become malnourished.

During hot weather, the child may become extremely exhausted due to the large amount of salt lost from the body in the perspiration. The preliminary diagnosis of CF is based on the high salt content of the sweat.

There is no single treatment and no cure for cystic fibrosis. The child is put on a daily regimen of antibiotics, pancreatic enzymes, and **vitamins.** The life expectancy for children with cystic fibrosis has been greatly increased in recent years.

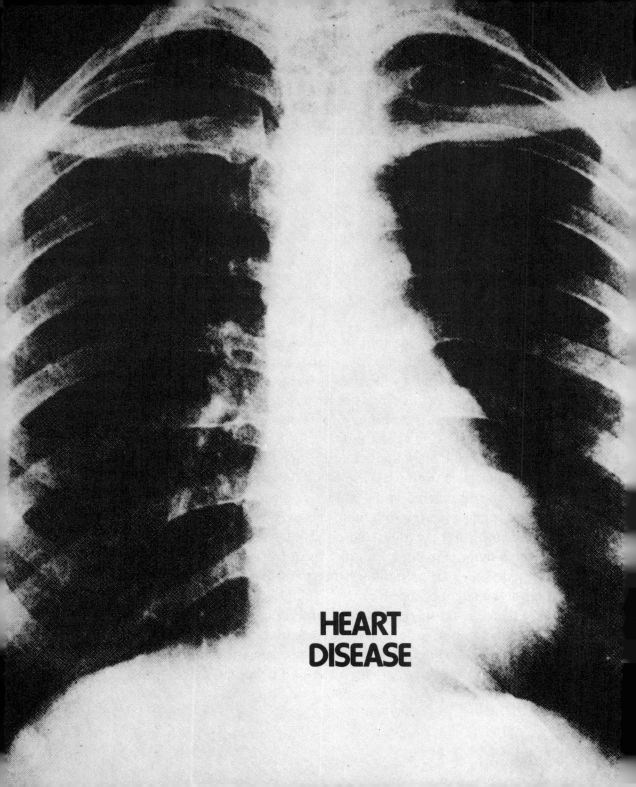

HEART
DISEASE

In the United States, two people die of heart disease every minute. It is the country's leading cause of death.

Heart disease is any disorder that interferes with the heart's ability to meet the continuous demands of the body. There are many different types of heart disease and many different causes. This is because the heart is such a complex **organ.** There may be a disorder of the specialized muscle tissue responsible for the pace at which the heart beats. There may be a disorder of the **valves,** the tiny flaps of tissue between the chambers of the heart that keep the blood flowing in the right direction. Or there may be a disorder in the **coronary arteries,** the small **arteries** that supply the heart muscle with blood.

CORONARY ARTERY DISEASE

Coronary artery disease (CAD) is by far the most common and life-threatening disease of the heart. It is the number-one killer in North America and Europe. It is the disease that causes heart attacks.

Of all the cases of CAD, 99 percent are caused by **athero-sclerosis.** Atherosclerosis is a condition in which blood vessels are narrowed by fat deposits along their inside walls, thus causing decreased blood flow. The name comes from two Greek words, **athere,** meaning "porridge" or "mush," and **scleros,** meaning "hard." The words describe how the fat deposits are soft in the beginning and then harden with age. Atherosclerosis may develop in any blood vessel, but it most often strikes the coronary arteries.

The most outstanding symptom of CAD is chest pain. Everyone feels chest pain of some type or other during his or her lifetime, but the pain from CAD is special. It is called **angina pectoris.** Some people describe it as a tight feeling behind the

Your Heart and How it Works

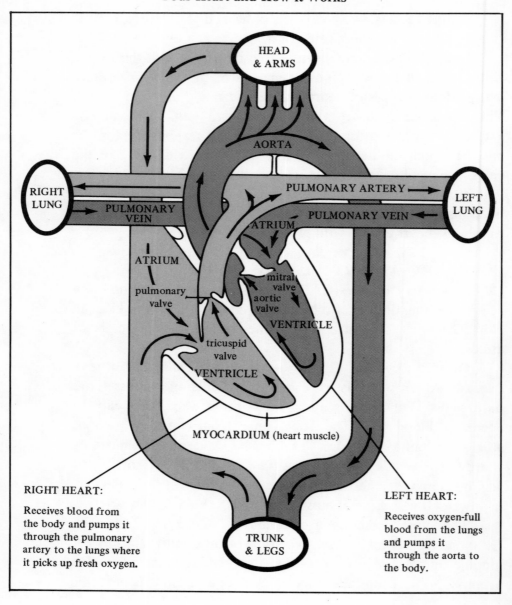

HEAD & ARMS

AORTA

RIGHT LUNG

PULMONARY VEIN

PULMONARY ARTERY

LEFT LUNG

PULMONARY VEIN

ATRIUM

ATRIUM

mitral valve

pulmonary valve

aortic valve

VENTRICLE

tricuspid valve

VENTRICLE

MYOCARDIUM (heart muscle)

RIGHT HEART:

Receives blood from the body and pumps it through the pulmonary artery to the lungs where it picks up fresh oxygen.

LEFT HEART:

Receives oxygen-full blood from the lungs and pumps it through the aorta to the body.

TRUNK & LEGS

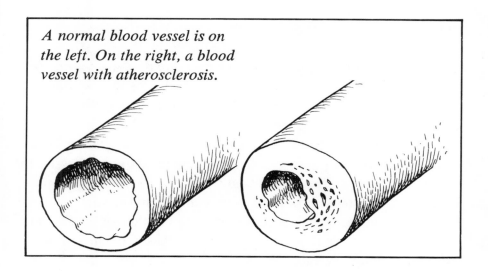

A normal blood vessel is on the left. On the right, a blood vessel with atherosclerosis.

breastbone. But it can also be described as a heavy or burning feeling and can be felt in the arms, jaws, or back. The pain is caused by an insufficient blood supply to part of the heart muscle. This decreased amount of blood may be enough for the heart muscle cells during normal activity. However, when the body is under increased **stress** during exercise, strong emotion, exposure to cold, or after a large meal, the heart needs a greater supply of oxygen, which it cannot get. This lack of oxygen, known as **hypoxia,** stimulates the nerve endings and thus, the sensation of pain.

The pain of angina only lasts about five minutes and rest helps to relieve it. Many people take medicine for the pain. The most common medicine used is **nitroglycerin.** This is in the form of small pills people dissolve under their tongues. This drug relaxes **smooth muscle.** Smooth muscle is the type of muscle found in the middle layer of the wall of the artery. It is also found in the other parts of the body, such as the walls of the intestines. A person has no conscious control over smooth muscle. The smooth muscle of the coronary artery is relaxed and expands, or dilates, as a result of the nitroglycerin. This allows the blood flow to increase, and the pain of angina goes away.

A more severe chest pain is that caused by a **heart attack.** This pain does not go away in a few minutes. It is not relieved by rest or nitroglycerin. The reason is that the blood flow has not been simply decreased, but has been completely blocked. It can be blocked in two ways: the fatty deposits of atherosclerosis can either get so thick as to completely clog the vessel, or the deposits can form a rough surface where blood clots can get stuck. Since the blood flow is stopped, the oxygen supply is stopped. The cells that were supplied by the blocked artery are damaged and will die. The damaged area interferes with the heart's ability to work efficiently. The whole heart is weakened and has trouble meeting the demands of the body. The person may perspire, have trouble breathing, feel nauseous, or vomit. The heart may be unable to contract effectively. This complication without medical help often leads to a quick death.

TREATMENT AND PREVENTION

With the many advances in medical know-how, death from heart attacks can be prevented. The most important goal of treatment is to keep the demands of the body at a minimum. This will reduce the workload of the heart. The heart is then able to mend itself. Tough scar tissue replaces the dead cells and surrounding blood vessels extend themselves and reroute the blood through the heart muscle. This is called **collateral circulation.** It is a very important facet of the heart's own built-in repair system. If the heart is allowed sufficient time to mend itself, it can do many more years of good work.

Sometimes, collateral circulation does not develop the way it should and the blocked artery will continue to cause trouble. Surgeons have developed an operation to prevent the threat of another attack. It is called **coronary artery bypass.** A vessel is taken from another part of the body and attached to the blocked artery to reroute the blood around the blockage. It is like a detour from a highway. These operations have been successful but no operation is without risk.

The big campaign, as in all disease, is on prevention. This is not so easy because doctors are not sure how to prevent atherosclerosis. Studies have outlined certain risk factors involved in the development of CAD. These are the amount of **cholesterol** in the diet, cigarette smoking, **obesity,** high blood pressure, diabetes, and sedentary and stressful occupations. Many people believe that if these factors are avoided, the chance of developing CAD is minimal.

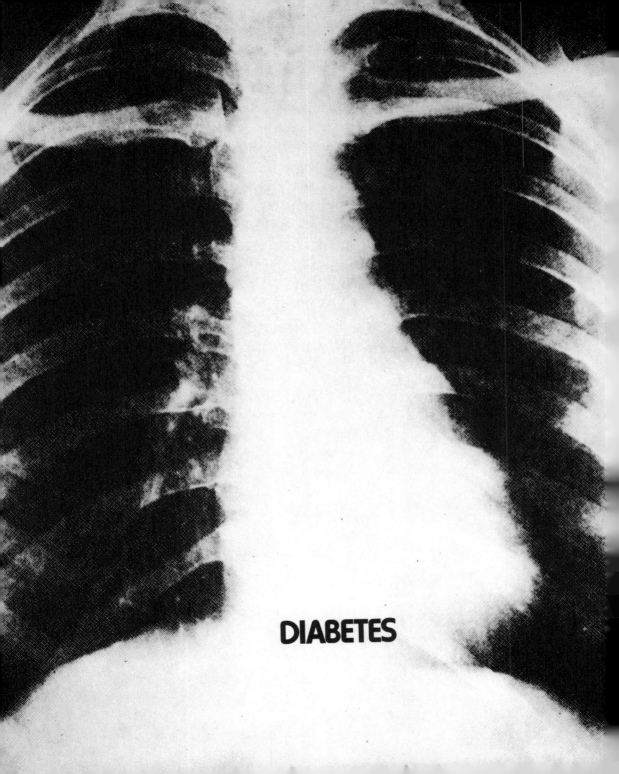

DIABETES

There are more than six million persons in the United States who have diabetes. In the United Kingdom there are probably 1,200,000 diabetics. It is one of the most widespread diseases. Diabetes is the leading cause of blindness occurring after birth, and diabetics are seventeen times more prone to kidney problems. The diabetic is twice as likely to develop heart disease.

The fact that a person with diabetes is called a diabetic may give you a clue that diabetes is a disease that affects the whole person. It is a disorder that affects the body's **metabolism,** specifically, **carbohydrate** metabolism. Metabolism is a general name for all the chemical processes that take place within the cells of the body. Carbohydrate metabolism refers to the way the cells use carbohydrates. The most important carbohydrate is **glucose.** Glucose is a sugar that is obtained by the body from the foods you eat, such as bread, cake, and potatoes. The cells metabolize glucose to get the energy needed for their work.

SYMPTOMS

Diabetes affects carbohydrate metabolism because of a problem in **insulin** production. Insulin is a **hormone** produced by the **beta cells** of the pancreas. The role of insulin is to help the glucose move into the cells from the blood. In children who have diabetes, there is no insulin production. This type is called juvenile diabetes. In adult onset diabetes, which people get when they are older, the insulin that is produced is inadequate in either amount or effectiveness. When there is not enough insulin, or no insulin at all, the glucose remains in the blood. The cells are then deprived of energy. This makes a person with diabetes feel weak. Even though the diabetic is taking in glucose by eating, the cells are not getting the glucose. It is not being used or stored by the

[33]

body. The kidneys attempt to clear the blood of this excess glucose by excretion in the urine. In order to excrete the glucose, the kidneys must dilute it with extra water. This process makes the diabetic urinate frequently. The diabetic also feels very thirsty because of all the water passed in the urine.

The cells then send messages to the brain that they need glucose. These messages cause the person to feel hungry. Soon the cells realize that even if the person eats more they can't use the glucose, so other energy sources are used. Fat deposits and protein stores can be broken down to provide energy. This causes the person to lose weight and feel tired. When fat deposits are broken down, acid by-products called **ketones** are released into the blood. This makes the blood too acidic.

The blood of a person with diabetes contains too much sugar and is too acidic. In some way this blood interferes with the way the body's white blood cells combat infection. Because of this, the diabetic often has a problem of slow-healing infections.

The abnormal thirst, the frequent urination, and the abnormal hunger are almost always symptoms of diabetes. The feeling of weakness, loss of weight, and slow-healing infections are sometimes symptoms of diabetes. Tests that show the amount of glucose in the blood and urine are used by the doctor to diagnose diabetes.

The cause of diabetes is unknown. It is believed to be inherited. This belief is due to the fact that people with diabetic parents and relatives run a high risk of developing diabetes. The exact way diabetes is inherited is not known. Besides genetic factors, there is a risk that older people, obese people, and women who have had many children will get diabetes. Diabetes is more likely to affect these groups of people possibly because the beta cells of their pancreases are overworked and become exhausted.

TREATMENT

There is no cure for diabetes but it can be controlled. The basic treatment for diabetes consists of balancing three factors: diet, exercise, and insulin medication. The diabetic learns to eat a balanced diet—the right foods in the right amounts at the right times. By keeping to this diet, the diabetic is able to keep his or her blood glucose level stable. Exercise has an insulin-like quality. It lowers the blood sugar level, thus decreasing the need for insulin. The third aspect of the treatment, insulin therapy, may or may not be needed. Many diabetics are able to control their diabetes by diet and exercise alone. But to many diabetics insulin is a lifesaver. Before 1922, the average life span of a diabetic was from five to ten years after the diagnosis was first made. In 1922 two Canadian scientists, Frederick Banting and Charles Best, isolated insulin from a dog pancreas. This discovery paved the way for the use of insulin from the pancreases of sheep, hogs, and cattle in the treatment of human diabetes. Insulin must be injected into the body with a needle. If it were taken orally, the stomach **enzymes** would destroy it.

There are also pills that can be given to lower blood sugar. These are called oral **hypoglycemics.** They work either by stimulating the beta cells to produce more insulin, or by somehow improving the functioning of the insulin. These pills can only be used by people who produce some insulin of their own. Juvenile diabetics are insulin dependent because they produce none of their own insulin.

When diabetes is not controlled, serious complications can result. Before the discovery of insulin, death was due to **acidosis.** Acidosis is too much acid in the blood. It occurs in diabetics when ketones build up in the blood. The excess acid affects the whole body and produces many symptoms, such as thirst, nausea, shortness of breath, and drowsiness. Acidosis can lead to coma and death. This condition can be corrected by giving the diabetic insulin.

Problems also arise when there is too much insulin. Too much insulin results in too little sugar in the blood. This can

Diabetics should carry Medic Alert cards in case of emergency.

MEDIC ALERT MEMBER INFORMATION	MEMBER NUMBER
SMITH, MARY JANE	6548369

7605 PARK AVE
NEW YORK, NY 11554
(212)634-1987
IN AN EMERGENCY CALL
DR THOMAS JOHNSON (212)687-1492
GERALD SMITH (212)634-1987
MY MEDICAL PROBLEM IS
DIABETES

)TAKES NPH U100 INSULIN, DIGOXIN
DATE ISSUED 6/10/76
IN AN EMERGENCY CALL COLLECT (209) 634-4917

happen if the diabetic takes too much medication, misses a meal, or performs heavy exercise. This condition is called **insulin shock.** Insulin shock can also produce different symptoms, such as weakness, hunger, blurred vision, abnormal actions, or sweating. A person in insulin shock can even appear to be drunk. Insulin shock is corrected by giving the diabetic glucose.

Both acidosis and insulin shock are medical emergencies. But they can be corrected. There are some complications that diabetics are prone to that cannot be corrected. These conditions take a long time to show up. For some reason, diabetes affects the blood vessels. In the large blood vessels, atherosclerosis may develop. The blood supply to the heart, brain, or feet can be decreased. This may cause coronary artery disease, **stroke,** or **gangrene** of the toes and feet. Gangrene is the death of tissue that occurs when the blood supply is cut off. If this occurs, the toes and feet will have to be amputated.

In the small blood vessels, **microangiopathy** can occur. Microangiopathy occurs when the small blood vessels thicken and then are destroyed. This condition only happens with diabetes. It is believed to be linked to the diabetic gene. The small blood vessels in the eyes and kidneys are most seriously affected. If these vessels are destroyed, blindness and kidney disease result.

Doctors are not sure how diabetes causes atherosclerosis and microangiopathy. There is an indication that if diabetes is controlled, these complications can be prevented or at least delayed.

Interestingly enough, a well-controlled diabetic can often be healthier than a nondiabetic. This is because a diabetic eats well, gets the right amount of exercise, and sees a doctor regularly.

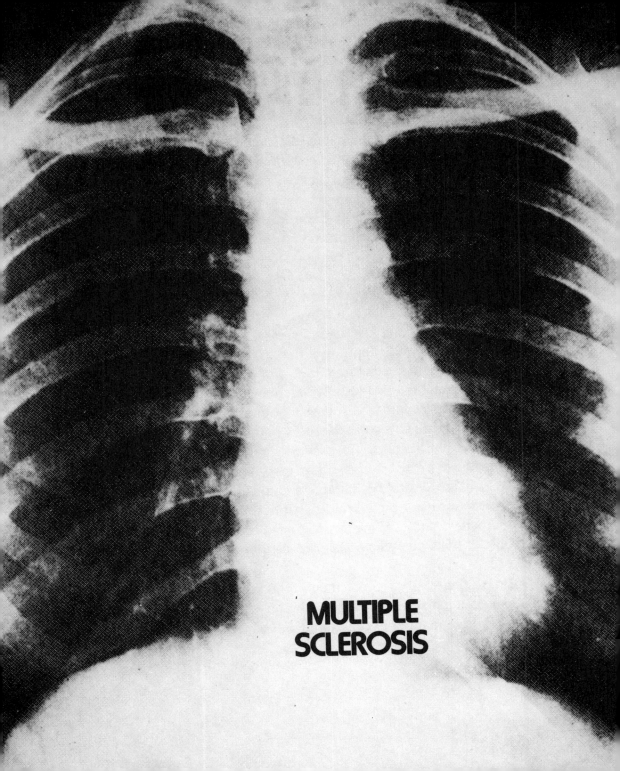

Multiple sclerosis usually strikes young adults between the ages of twenty and forty. Multiple sclerosis (MS) is a disease of the nervous system. The cause is unknown. It can affect any area of the central nervous system. There are a variety of symptoms.

In the body, the nerves are covered with fatty tissue called the **myelin sheath.** The myelin sheath helps the passage of impulses along the nerves. It allows the nerve impulse to travel faster and also nourishes the nerve material itself. In multiple sclerosis, the myelin sheath breaks down leaving patches of exposed nerve. Tough scar tissue covers these patches, but nerve impulses have trouble getting past these hard spots.

If the myelin sheath of the spinal cord is affected, the person may suffer from weakness, lack of coordination, or paralysis of the trunk, hands, and feet. If different parts of the brain are affected, the symptoms may be the loss of balance, slurred speech, double vision, or emotional disturbances. These are only a few of the symptoms. There are many more.

Strangely, the symptoms usually last only a few weeks, and the person seems to recover. At any time, though, the symptoms may reappear. Sometimes they may stay away for years. This "go away" and "come back" pattern is characteristic of the disease. The way MS shows itself varies from person to person. Also, there is no test to prove that a person has MS.

Another baffling aspect of MS is that the closer the person lives to the equator, the less risk the person runs of developing the disease. This is called **geographic distribution.** It means that people living in a certain part of the world are more prone to a certain disease. There are more cases of MS in populations that live more than 40° north or south of the equator than in popula-

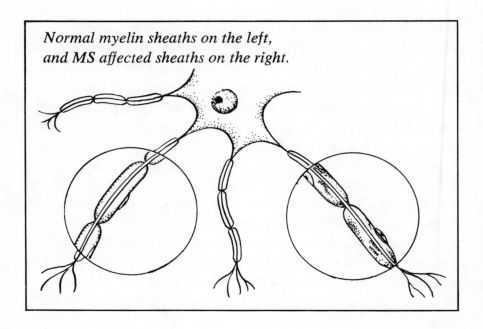

*Normal myelin sheaths on the left,
and MS affected sheaths on the right.*

tions that live near the equator. Because of this geographic distribution, scientists think that something in the environment may
cause MS.

MS DISEASE THEORIES

Regarding the cause of the disease, there are three theories under
heavy investigation. One is that the disease is caused by a slow-
acting virus. This virus might infect the body early in a person's
life, but then take years to produce damage. The virus may be the
rubella (measles) virus, or it may be linked with it. There is also
a theory that the MS virus is carried by dogs, and may be trans-

mitted through the dogs' urine. The virus could be de-activated by sunlight and this would account for the prevalence of MS in areas of less sunlight, that is, farther away from the equator.

Another theory is that MS is an **autoimmune disease.** For some reason antibodies recognize the myelin sheath as foreign and attack it by mistake. The third theory combines the two other theories. Some researchers think that some viral agent triggers an autoimmune response.

TREATMENT

Treatment for MS depends upon the case. The main emphasis is on keeping the person in otherwise good health. Preventing infection, maintaining a good diet, and getting plenty of rest are important goals of treatment. Physical therapy, surgery, and chemotherapy are sometimes used. As of yet there is no cure. But the picture is not as bleak as many people think. One doctor finds that for every MS patient that comes into his office in a wheel-chair, four MS patients come in walking. The life span of a person with MS is not really any shorter than for a person who does not have MS.

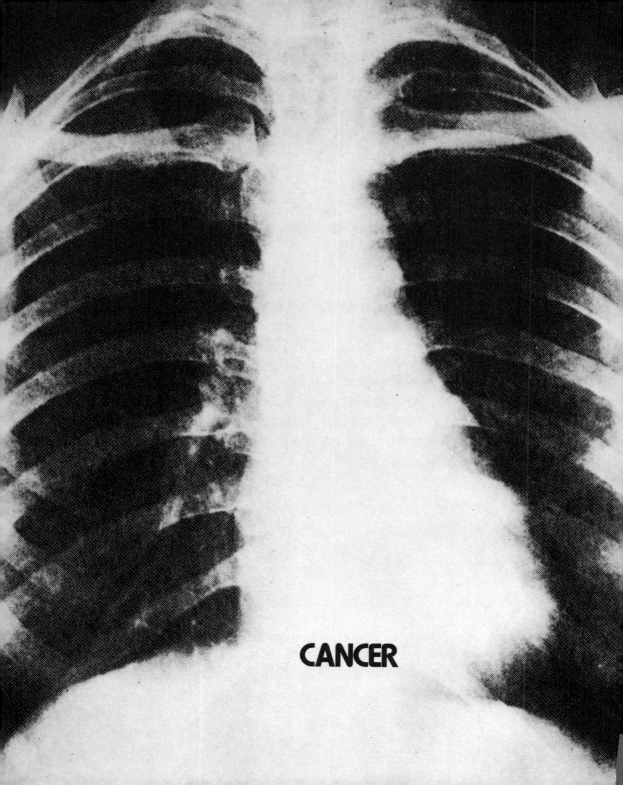

Among the diseases that plague humanity today, there is none so dread as cancer. One out of every four people have or will develop cancer. Although the number of cases of cancer seems to be increasing in these modern times, cancer may be the most ancient of diseases. In the fifth century B.C., Hippocrates used the Greek word for "crab" to describe this disease. "Cancer" is the Latin word for crab. It got its name from the way that cancerous growths are like pincers that choke the life out of healthy tissue.

WHAT ARE CANCERS?

Cancer is not one disease but many—about 150 types have been identified in humans. Each type is defined by the kind of cell and the part of the body in which it is found. There are two main groups. First, the **carcinomas** that are found in the **epithelial tissue,** that is, the lining tissue of the throat, lungs, stomach, glands, and so forth. Carcinomas account for about 85 percent of human cancers. The second group is called the **sarcomas.** These cancers invade the bones, muscles, cartilage, tendons, blood, and the reproductive organs. Two large subgroups of the sarcomas are the **leukemias** and the **lymphomas.** Leukemia is a cancer in which abnormal **leukocytes** (white blood cells) accumulate in the blood and bone marrow. Lymphoma is a disease in which abnormal numbers of **lymphocytes** (another type of white blood cell) are produced by the spleen and **lymph nodes.** Hodgkin's disease is the best-known form of lymphoma.

All of these forms of cancer have one thing in common. They represent the runaway growth of abnormal body cells. The seriousness of the disease in each person depends upon the site of growth and how rapidly the cancer cells are dividing and spreading. Every cancer begins as a single abnormal cell that

[43]

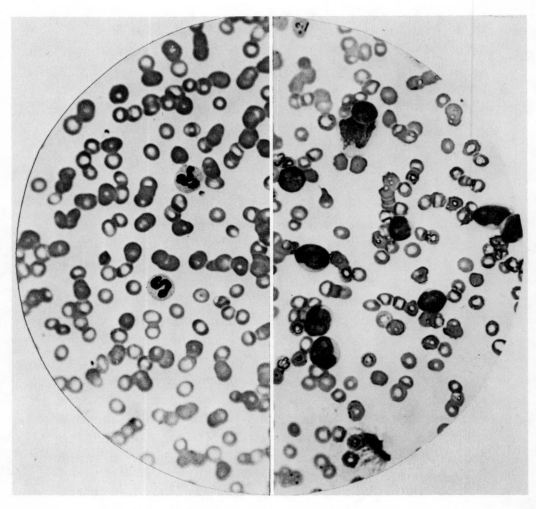

On the left, normal blood with
two white blood cells. On the right,
leukemia is indicated by five
times the number of white blood cells.

seems to have blocked itself off from any of the body's normal controls. One of the normal controls is **contact inhibition.** This means that the pressure of one cell against another inhibits, or stops, further cell division in that area. With cancer cells, however, no such control is present.

BENIGN TUMOROUS GROWTHS AND
MALIGNANT TUMOROUS GROWTHS

It is important to distinguish cancerous growths or **malignant tumorous growths** from noncancerous growths or **benign tumorous growths.** The word benign comes from the Latin *bene* meaning "good" and *genus* which means "sort." Thus a benign tumorous growth is a "good sort of **tumorous growth.**" It is good in the sense that it is a tumorous growth of slow, limited growth that remains in one part of the body. It will not radically harm or kill its host, unless it becomes large enough to interfere mechanically with surrounding structures. It can easily be removed in most cases. Malignant tumorous growths, on the other hand, represent a serious threat to the life and well-being of the host. The word malignant comes from the Latin word *malus,* which means "bad." This is the "bad sort of tumorous growth" that grows in a wild, disorganized fashion. These tumorous growths invade surrounding tissues, drawing off nutrients from them. Worst of all, malignant tumorous growths release cancer cells into the **lymph fluid** and the blood. These cells are then carried to tissue in other parts of the body where they may start new sites of malignant growth. This spreading of dislodged cancer cells is called **metastasis.**

Metastasis is the most lethal aspect of the disease of cancer. There are three factors that seem to play a part in the ability of cancer cells to metastasize. One, cancer cells have a lower co-

[45]

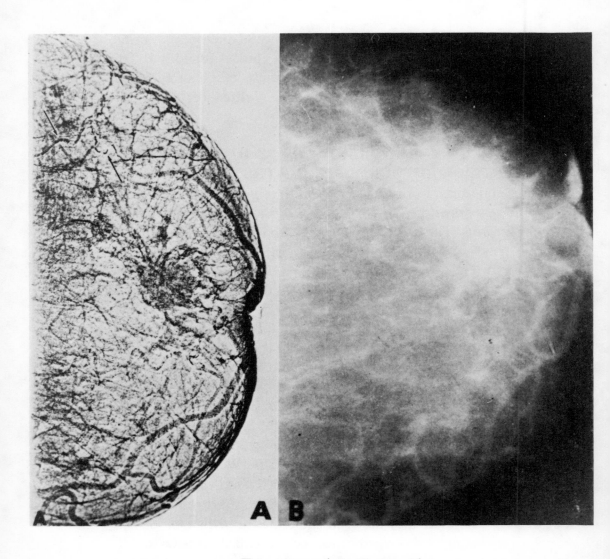

*Two views of carcinoma of
the breast, indicated by
thickened areas in both cases.*

hesiveness, or sticking action, than normal cells, and this allows them to break away. Two, cancer cells have the ability to survive for a period of time independent of other cells. Three, cancer cells are able to invade normal tissue and grow there.

SYMPTOMS AND TREATMENT
The early stages of malignant growths produce no symptoms. This is a problem because it is only when the growth has reached a later and more dangerous stage of development that cancer shows itself to the victim. The common warning signs are fatigue, change in bowel habits, sores that don't seem to heal, rapid loss of weight, a lump or thickening on the body, unusual bleeding or discharge, indigestion or difficulty in swallowing, or an obvious change in a wart or a mole.

If cancer can be detected early enough, the chances for the complete elimination of the cancerous growth are good. This is done through surgery, chemicals, hormones, **radiation therapy,** or a combination of these. The last three are effective because they interfere with or destroy rapidly dividing cells in the body. But they also destroy certain healthy cells as well.

WHAT CAUSES CANCER?
No one factor can be pinpointed as being the cause of the various types of cancerous growths. Some progress has been made in isolating factors—present in significant numbers—that have a definite effect in cancer formation. Environmental factors lead the list. Harmful elements in the air you breathe (including cigarette smoke), the food you eat, and the water you drink may all contribute to the possibility of cancer. Radiation has been shown to cause cancer. Radiation can be both helpful and harmful. Ra-

diation therapy can destroy cancerous tissue, as mentioned above. Uncontrolled radiation, however, can change the genetic structure of healthy cells and cause them to become cancerous. Viruses have been proven to cause certain cancers in animals. It is highly probable that viruses may cause certain human cancers as well. Although people don't seem to "catch" the cancer virus from a diseased person, a virus can still be a cause of cancer.

One theory explains that perhaps an inactive cancer virus is present in each and every body cell. It could have been a part of the DNA long before complex organisms developed on the earth. When for whatever reason this virus is activated, it changes the normal cell into a cancerous cell.

Related to the viral factors are the genetic factors. There is a current theory that cancerous cells arise spontaneously as **mutations** (a change in a cell's DNA). Mutations occur all of the time among all rapidly dividing cells. In most of the cases, these mutant cells are quickly wiped out by the body's immune system. The reason why certain people do develop cancer, the theory runs, is because of some defect in their system of immune response. For some reason, the cancer cells are not recognized as abnormal or foreign by the antibodies. Something further could be at stake here. It could be that these cancer cells secrete an enzyme of some sort that retards or stops the immune reaction.

There are three areas of evidence that support the theory that the immune system has an important effect on cancer. First, older adults are more likely to get cancer. Some scientists believe that this is because the immune system becomes less active as a person gets older. Second, cancer spreads more rapidly in patients who are on drugs that suppress the immune system. Third, in some people the cancers, even "incurable" cancers, have spontaneously become smaller and have even totally disappeared. It may be that the body's immune system started to attack the cancer in these cases. If researchers could learn the secret of what triggered this spontaneous **remission,** they could use the same process to rid a body of cancer.

Whatever the causal factors of cancer, the question posed by most cancer research today is, "What is it that changes a normal body cell into a cancer cell?" Some of the researchers are studying and experimenting with the normal process of **cell differentiation.** You began life as a single cell, yet are now a complex organism composed of millions of specialized cells. How do cells become different? This is one of the unsolved mysteries of science. The more scientists learn about this process, the more they will know about how a cell becomes cancerous.

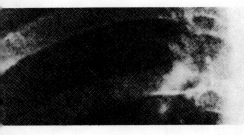

GLOSSARY

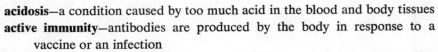

acidosis—a condition caused by too much acid in the blood and body tissues

active immunity—antibodies are produced by the body in response to a vaccine or an infection

anemia—a symptom of many diseases, in which there is something lacking in the blood, such as red blood cells

angina pectoris—sudden pain in the chest caused by interference with the supply of oxygen to the heart

antibiotic—a chemical compound used to stop the growth or the life of disease-producing organisms

antibody—a protein made in the body in response to an antigen; the antibody binds itself to the antigen to overcome the toxic effects of the antigen

antibody-antigen complex—the union of an antibody and an antigen

antigen—any substance not normally present in the body, such as a virus, which causes antibodies to be made

artery—a blood vessel that carries blood away from the heart to other parts of the body

atherosclerosis—the buildup of fatty material on the inside wall of an artery

autoimmune disease—a disease caused by one's own cells or antibodies attacking one's own body tissues

bacteria—microscopic organisms that are found everywhere and may be helpful or harmful to other living things

benign tumorous growth—a growth that usually does not endanger life, because it does not invade surrounding tissue

beta cells—special cells in the pancreas that make insulin

black death—a name given to the plague that spread through Europe during the fourteenth century. The plague is a highly fatal disease caused by bacteria. It is carried by rats and spread to humans by their fleas. Because black spots may appear on the body during the course of the disease, it was called the black death.

cancer—disease characterized by the uncontrolled proliferation of abnormal body cells

carbohydrate—a compound of carbon, hydrogen, and oxygen found in most foods and an important source of energy for the body

carcinoma—a malignant tumorous growth found in epithelial tissue

carriers—persons who can spread disease to others even though they are not affected by the disease themselves

cell differentiation—the process by which a cell is changed in structure to perform a specific function

central nervous system—that portion of the nervous system consisting of the brain and spinal cord

chancre—the painless sore that appears in the first stage of syphilis

cholesterol—a sterol ($C_{27}H_{45}OH$) that occurs in all animal fats

chromosome—a threadlike structure composed mostly of DNA; it is found in the nucleus of the cell and contains genes

chronic—lasting a long time

collateral circulation—the opening of smaller arteries to supply blood to an area where a larger artery is closed or narrowed

coma—a state of prolonged unconsciousness due to disease or injury

complement—proteins that bind to the antibody-antigen complex and destroy a foreign invader

contact inhibition—a normal control of cell growth, whereby the pressure of one cell against another inhibits, or stops, further cell division in that area

contagious—spread easily from one person to another

coronary arteries—the arteries that supply the heart muscle with blood

coronary artery bypass—a heart operation that reroutes the blood through a transplanted artery

coronary artery disease—a disease of the heart caused by a blockage of the coronary arteries

cowpox—a viral infection found in cattle and related to smallpox in humans

cystic fibrosis—a genetic disease caused by a recessive gene affecting different glands of the body

diabetes—a disorder of carbohydrate metabolism, whereby the blood sugar level is elevated because of a problem in insulin production

diphtheria—a highly contagious childhood disease caused by a bacteria that infects the throat

DNA—deoxyribonucleic acid, a large complex molecule that is the basic substance of genes

dominant gene—a strong trait that does not require the presence of a pair to appear in an organism

enzymes—substances found in the body that speed up or slow down chemical changes

epidemic—spreading rapidly and affecting many people

epithelial tissue—the cells that line the inside and outside surfaces of the body

gangrene—the death and rotting of body tissue, caused by the stoppage of blood supply

genes—the units of hereditary traits that are found in the chromosomes of each cell

genetics—the scientific study of hereditary traits pertaining to the genes or traits that are inherited from one's parents

genital area—the location of the organs involved in reproduction

geographic distribution—the spread of a disease through a certain area of the earth

germs—microscopic organisms that can cause infections

glucose—a simple sugar that is the most important source of the body's energy

gonococcus—a round bacterium that causes gonorrhea

gonorrhea—the most common venereal disease

gumma—sores that appear in the third stage of syphilis

heart attack—the sudden cutoff of blood to an area of the heart muscle, resulting in muscle tissue death

heart disease—a general term given to any disorder that affects the function of the heart

hemoglobin—the oxygen-carrying molecule found in the red blood cells

hepatitis—inflammation of the liver, usually due to a virus infection in the blood

heredity—the transmission of traits from parents to offspring

hormone—a chemical secretion of a ductless gland that produces a definite effect in the body

hydrophobia—another name for rabies; the term refers to the infected person's intense fear of water during the second stage of rabies

hypoxia—a general term meaning the lack of oxygen supply to the body tissues

hypoglycemics—drugs that lower the blood sugar level

immune system—the complex system that protects the body from disease

immunity—resistance to a disease

incubation period—the time between exposure to infectious disease and the appearance of symptoms

infection—invasion of the body by a harmful organism

infectious disease—a disease caused by infection

inflammation—localized heat, redness, swelling, and pain due to injury or infection

inoculation—the introduction of harmful organisms into the body to start the production of antibodies

insulin—a hormone made in the pancreas that helps move glucose from the blood into the cells

insulin shock—a condition caused by too much insulin in the blood resulting in a dangerously low level of sugar in the blood

ketones—an acidic by-product resulting from the breakdown of fat deposits

latent—present but hidden; the latent stage of a disease is a time when the disease is still present but there are no symptoms

leukemia—a cancer in which abnormal leukocytes accumulate in the blood and bone marrow

leukocytes—white blood cells

lymph fluid—the clear liquid part of the blood that circulates in the lymph vessels

lymph nodes—enlargements in the lymph vessels that act as filters for lymph fluid

lymphocytes—a type of white blood cell that is smaller than other white blood cells and has a round nucleus

lymphoma—a cancer in which abnormal numbers of lymphocytes are produced by the spleen and lymph nodes; Hodgkin's disease is the best-known form of lymphoma

malignant tumorous growth—a growth that invades surrounding tissues and may spread to other parts of the body; it can be fatal

measles—a highly contagious illness caused by a virus, measles is marked by a red rash that covers the body

metabolism—a general term for the chemical processes that take place within the body

metastasis—the spread of disease from one part of the body to another part by way of the blood, the lymph fluid, or membranous surfaces

microangiopathy—a disorder, sometimes found in diabetics, in which there is destruction of small blood vessels

microbe—a microorganism; an animal or plant that can only be seen with the aid of a microscope

mucous membrane—the lining of the inner surfaces of the body; it contains glands that secrete the thick fluid called mucus

multiple sclerosis—a disease of the nervous system marked by hard patches in the brain and spinal cord

mumps—a viral disease that attacks the largest pair of salivary glands, the parotid glands, causing the swelling under the jawbone

mutation—a change in a cell's DNA

myelin sheath—the fatty coating around certain nerves

nitroglycerin—a chemical that is used to relieve the chest pains of angina pectoris by expanding the blood vessels; it is also used as an explosive

noninfectious disease—a disease that is not caused by any infectious organism

obesity—the condition of being overweight

organ—a group of tissues that work together to perform a special job or function in the body

organism—any living being, plant, or animal

pancreas—a large organ located below the stomach that makes both enzymes and hormones

paralysis—loss of the ability to move parts of the body

passive immunity—transfer into the individual of antibodies that have been produced in other individuals or animals

pelvic organs—those organs supported by the bowl-shaped skeletal structure formed by the hip bones and the lower part of the vertebral column

penicillin—an antibiotic

polio—poliomyelitis; a contagious viral disease that attacks the central nervous system causing paralysis; also called infantile paralysis

protein—a complex compound found in all living matter and necessary for the growth and repair of living tissue

pus—collection of dead bacteria and white blood cells at the site of an infection

rabies—a fatal viral infection that attacks the central nervous system; it is spread to humans by the bite of an infected mammal

radiation therapy—the use of X rays or radioactive substances to destroy living cells, such as cancer cells

recessive gene—a weak trait that requires the presence of its pair to physically appear in an organism

remission—improvement or disappearance of the symptoms of a disease

rubella—a mild viral disease, dangerous to pregnant women since the virus can damage the baby; also called German measles

sarcoma—any of various malignant tumorous growths that are found in connective tissue, especially bones and muscles

serum—the clear, pale yellow liquid that separates from the clot in the coagulation of blood; it contains antibodies

sickle cell disease—a genetic disease, caused by a recessive gene, that causes red blood cells to assume a sickled shape in the event of limited oxygen

sickle cell trait—the condition of carrying only one of the pair of recessive genes for sickle cell disease in the body cells; usually no symptoms of the disease are present in the carrier, but the disease may be passed on to the carrier's offspring

smallpox—a serious contagious disease caused by a virus and marked by fever and skin eruptions

smooth muscle—the involuntary muscle that is found lining the walls of the intestines, stomach, and arteries

spirochete—a spiral-shaped bacterium

stress—any condition that causes strain or tension

stroke—the sudden cutoff of blood supply to an area in the brain

swine flu—an infection that is caused by a certain type of virus; this disease reached epidemic proportions in the first quarter of the twentieth century

symptom—a change in the person's normal state; it is an indication that something is wrong

syphilis—a venereal disease caused by a spirochete that can become very serious if untreated

Tay-Sachs disease—a genetic disease caused by a recessive gene whereby fatty material builds up in nerve cells and destroys them; it leads to death within a few years

tetanus—a fatal disease caused by bacteria; the first symptom is stiffness of the jaw, called lockjaw; the bacteria that cause it are found in the soil and most often enter humans through puncture wounds

tetracycline—an antibiotic effective against many microorganisms

tissue—a group of similar cells that perform a special task

trait—a distinguishing feature

tumorous growth—a swelling or enlargement due to abnormal overgrowth of tissue; it may be malignant or benign

vaccination—inoculation with dead or weakened microorganisms to prevent disease

vaccine—the dead or weakened or similar microorganisms that are used in a vaccination

valve—a fold of tissue that prevents fluids from flowing backwards

venereal disease—a disease that is spread from an infected person to another person through sexual contact

viral—caused by a virus

virus—tiny infectious agents that can reproduce only in living cells

vitamins—an organic substance that is essential for normal body activity

whooping cough—an infectious disease marked by violent attacks of coughing and vomiting; it is also called pertussis after the organism that causes it

World Health Organization (WHO)—the agency of the United Nations that is involved with the health of all nations

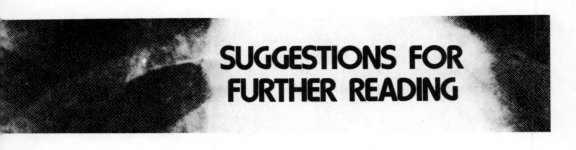

SUGGESTIONS FOR FURTHER READING

Aylesworth, Thomas G. *The World of Microbes*. (Collins Pub. International Library) New York: Franklin Watts, 1975.

Bedischi, Giulio. *Science of Medicine*. (Collins Pub.) New York: Franklin Watts, 1975.

Brown, J. A. C. (revised Hastin Bennett, M. A.), *Pears Medical Encyclopaedia*. London: Pelham, 1977.

Calder, Ritchie. *The Wonderful World of Medicine*. Garden City, New York: Doubleday, 1969.

Curtis, Robert H. *Medical Talk for Beginners*. New York: Julian Messner, 1976.

Gordon, Sol. *Facts About VD*. New York: John Day, 1973.

Kaplan, Colin (ed.). *Rabies: The Facts*. Oxford: Oxford University Press, 1977.

Knight, David C. *Your Body's Defenses*. New York: McGraw-Hill, 1975.

Nourse, Alan E. *Lumps, Bumps, and Rashes: A Look at Kid's Diseases*. New York: Franklin Watts, 1976.

————— *Viruses*. New York: Franklin Watts, 1976.

Simon, Tony. *The Heart Explorers*. New York: Basic Books, 1966.

For further information in the United States and Canada, the following organizations publish pamphlets:

The American Cancer Society, Inc.
209 East 42 Street
New York, New York 10017

American Diabetes Association, Inc.
18 East 48 Street
New York, New York 10017

American Heart Association
44 East 23 Street
New York, New York 10010

Center for Disease Control
Communicable Disease Center
Public Health Service
Atlanta, Georgia 30333

National Cystic Fibrosis Research Foundation
3379 Peachtree Road, N.E.
Atlanta, Georgia 30326

The National Foundation—March of Dimes
P.O. Box 2000
White Plains, New York 10602

National Multiple Sclerosis Society
205 East 42 Street
New York, New York 10017

United States Department of Health, Education and Welfare
U.S. Government Printing Office
Division of Public Documents
Washington, D.C. 20025

For further information in the United Kingdom, write to:

British Diabetic Association
3–6 Alfred Place
London, W.C. 1

British Heart Foundation
57 Gloucester Place
London, W. 1

Cancer Research Campaign
2 Carlton House Terrace
London, S.W. 1

Cystic Fibrosis Research Foundation Trust
5 Blyth Road
Bromley, Kent

Department of Health and Social Security
Alexander Fleming House
Elephant and Castle
London, S.E. 1

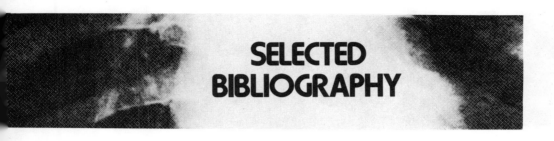

SELECTED BIBLIOGRAPHY

Apgar, Virginia, and Beck, Joan. *Is My Baby All Right? A Guide to Birth Defects.* New York: Trident Press, 1972.

Beadle, George, and Beadle, Muriel. *The Language of Life: An Introduction to the Science of Genetics.* Garden City, New York: Doubleday, 1966.

DeKruif, Paul. *Microbe Hunters.* New York: Harcourt, Brace and World, 1953.

Glasser, Ronald. *The Body Is the Hero.* New York: Random House, 1976.

Goodfield, June. *The Siege of Cancer.* New York: Random House, 1975.

Maugh, Thomas H., and Marx, Jean L. *Seeds of Destruction: The Science Report on Cancer Research.* New York: Plenum Press, 1975.

Miller, Benjamin F., and Keane, Clare Brackman. *Encyclopedia and Dictionary of Medicine and Nursing.* Philadelphia: W. B. Saunders Co., 1972.

Rosebury, Theodor. *Microbes and Morals: The Story of Venereal Disease.* New York: The Viking Press, 1971.

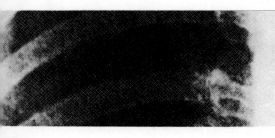

INDEX

Chromosomes, 20, 51
Chronic, defined, 51
Cigarette smoking, 31, 47
Collateral circulation, 30, 51
Coma, 12, 51
Complement, 7, 51
Contact inhibition, 45, 51
Contagious, defined, 51
Coronary artery, 27, 31, 51
Coronary artery bypass, 31, 51
Coronary artery disease, 27, 51
Cowpox, 5, 52
Cystic fibrosis, 25, 52

Deoxyribonucleic acid (DNA), 20, 48, 52
Diabetes, 52
    juvenile, 33, 35
    symptoms, 33–34
    treatment, 35–37
Digestion, 25
Diphtheria, 8, 52
Disease
    infectious, 2
    latent, 17
    noninfectious, 2, 54
DNA, 20, 48, 52
Dominant gene, 21, 52

Emotional disturbance, 39
Enyzmes, 35, 52
Epidemic, 3, 52
Epithelial tissue, 43

Flushing, 2

Gangrene, 37, 52
Genes, 20, 52
Genetic disease, 20,–25
Genetics, 20, 48, 52
Genitals, 15, 18, 52
Geographic distribution, 39
German measles, 8, 55
Germs, 2, 52
Glands, 25, 43
Glucose, 33–34, 52
Gonococcus, 15, 52
Gonorrhea, 15–18, 52
Gumma, 17, 52

Heart attack, 27, 30, 52
Heart disease, 27–31, 52
Heart muscle, 29–31
Hemoglobin, 22, 53
Hepatitis, 8, 53
Heredity, 20, 53
Hippocrates, 43
Hodgkin's disease, 43
Hormones, 33, 47, 53
Hydrophobia, 12, 53
Hypoglycemics, 35, 53
Hypoxia, 29, 53

Immune system, 7–8, 48, 53
Immunity, 53
    active, 7
    passive, 8
Incubation period, 10, 53
Infection, defined, 53
Infectious diseases, 2, 53
Inflammation, defined, 53

Inoculation, 5, 53
Insulin, 33, 35, 36, 53
Insulin shock, 37, 53
Iran, 13

Jenner, Edward, 5

Ketones, 34, 53
Kidneys, 23, 33, 37

Latent, defined, 53
Leukemia, 43, 53
Leukocytes, 43, 53
Liver, 8, 23
Lungs, 23
    cystic fibrosis, 25
Lymph fluid, 45, 53
Lymph nodes, 43, 53
Lymphocytes, 43, 54
Lymphoma, 43, 54

Malignant tumorous growths, 45, 54
Mammals, carriers of disease, 10–13
Measles, 8, 40, 54
Mental retardation, 25
Metabolism, 33, 54
Metastasis, 45, 54
Microangiopathy, 37, 54
Microbes, 15, 54
Moles, 47
Mucous membranes, 17, 54
Multiple sclerosis, 3, 39–43, 54
Mumps, 8, 54
Muscle, smooth, 29–30
Mutation, 20, 48, 54

Myelin sheath, 39, 54

Nervous system, 10, 39
Nitroglycerin, 29, 54
Noninfectious disease, 2, 54

Obesity, 31, 54
Organ, defined, 54
Organism, defined, 54

Pancreas, 25, 54
Paralysis, 8, 39, 55
Passive immunity, 8, 55
Pasteur, Louis, 5, 10
Pelvic organs, 55
Penicillin, 18, 55
Pertussis, 8
Physical therapy, 41
Polio, 8, 55
Pregnancy, and syphilis, 15
Proteins, 7, 55
Pus, 5, 55

Rabies, 2, 10–13, 55
Radiation, 47
Radiation therapy, 47, 55
Rash, 2
Recessive gene, 21, 55
Red blood cells, 22, 23
Remission, 48, 55
Reproductive organs, 43
Respiratory infections, 25
Rubella, 8, 40, 55
Rubeola, 8

Saliva, 10
Sarcoma, 43, 55
Scar tissue, 30
Serum, 8, 55
Sickle cell disease, 20, 22–23, 55
Sickle cell trait, 21, 55
Smallpox, 2, 5–8, 55
Smooth muscle, 29, 56
Spinal cord, 39
Spirochete, 15, 56
Spleen, 43
Sterility, 18
Stomach, 43
Stress, 56
Stroke, 37, 56
Surgery, 41
Sweat glands, 25
Swelling, 2
Swine flu, 8, 56
Symptom, defined, 56
Syphilis, 15–18, 56

Tay-Sachs disease, 23–25, 56

Tendons, 43
Tetanus, 8, 56
Tetracycline, 18, 56
Tissue, 56
Traits, 20, 56
Tumorous growths, 45, 56

United Kingdom, 5, 13, 33

Vaccination, 5, 7–8, 56
Vaccine, defined, 56
Valve, 56
Venereal disease, 3, 15–18, 56
Viral diseases, 8, 56
Virus, 2, 56
Vitamins, 25, 56

Warts, 47
Weight loss, 2, 34, 47
White blood cells, 7, 43
Whooping cough, 8, 56
World Health Organization, 5, 56

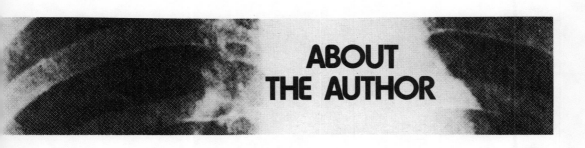

ABOUT THE AUTHOR

Marianne and Mary-Alice Tully, two of a family of eleven children, are free-lance science writers for children and pursue related fields. Mary-Alice has a B.S. degree in biology from Stony
Brook University, and is a registered nurse at Children's Hospital
Medical Center in Boston, Massachusetts. Marianne received a
master's degree from Hunter College, and is presently a teacher-
director of a Montessori school in New York City. Marianne
and Mary-Alice Tully are the authors of *Facts About the Human
Body* (A First Book) published by Franklin Watts.